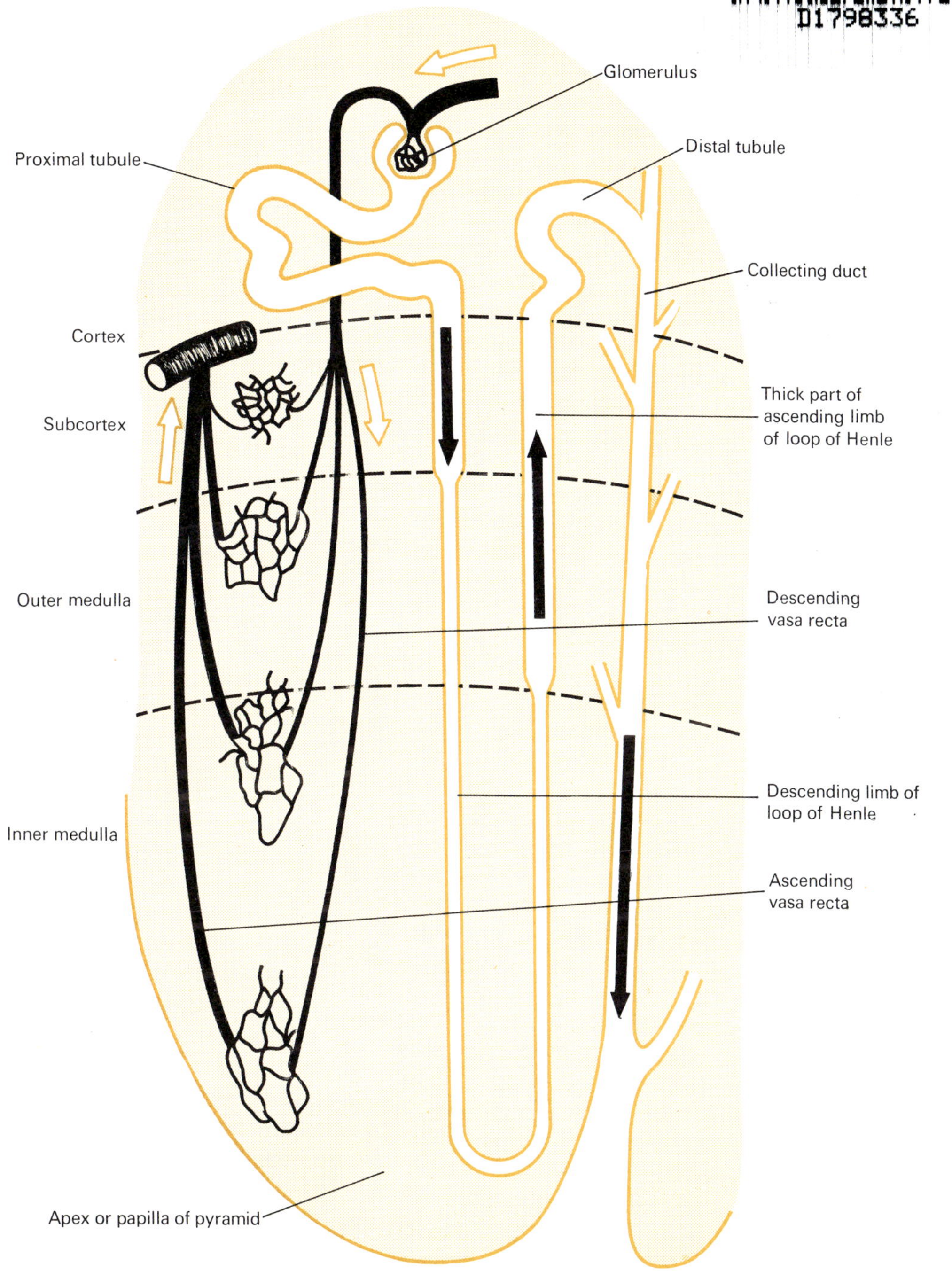

Glomerulus

Proximal tubule

Distal tubule

Collecting duct

Cortex

Subcortex

Thick part of
ascending limb
of loop of Henle

Outer medulla

Descending
vasa recta

Inner medulla

Descending limb of
loop of Henle

Ascending
vasa recta

Apex or papilla of pyramid

FIG. 1. Diagram (not to scale) to illustrate the portions of the nephron and the zones of the kidney in which they are found. White arrows indicate direction of blood flow; black arrows, flow of filtrate.

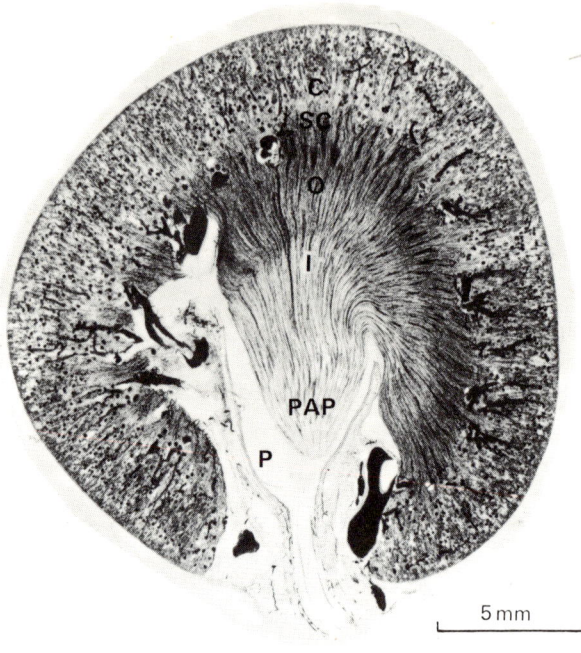

5 mm

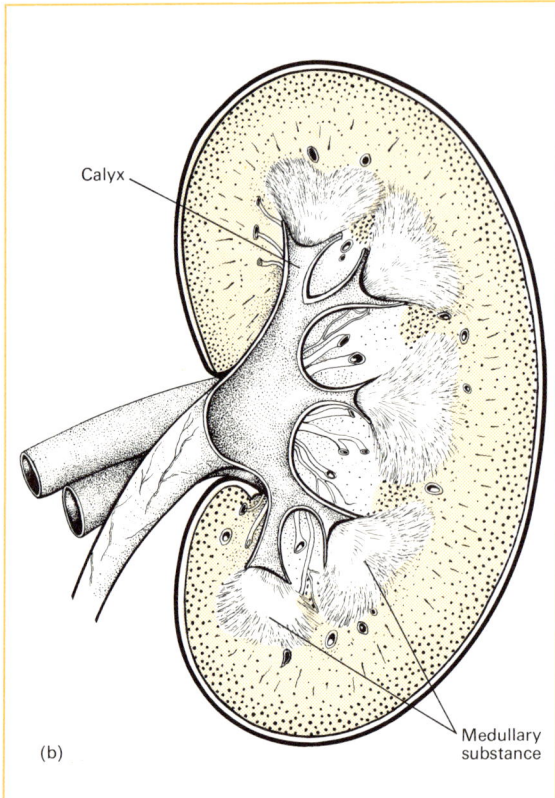

Calyx

Medullary
substance

(b)

The kidney has a number of functions which include the excretion of waste products and the regulation of the chemical composition and the acid–base balance of the body tissues. Perhaps its most obvious and familiar function, however, is its ability to maintain at a constant level the water content of the body and thus the osmotic environment of the tissues. For many years the kidney was regarded as nothing more than a complex filter in which the glomeruli produced a filtrate from the blood plasma which was modified as it passed along the tubules by the variable reabsorption of water and other substances and also by excretion into the tubular lumen. On this basis it was easy to understand the everyday observation that if one drinks a large quantity of water the kidneys produce a great deal of pale almost colourless urine, while on a hot, thirsty day the urine is darker in colour and is passed only in small quantities. Certain experimental findings, which will be mentioned later, made the original idea of kidney function untenable but it is only relatively recently that an alternative theory has been put forward as a result of the evidence produced by modern techniques.

Before describing the process of the production of urine by the kidney, it will be helpful to introduce the concept of *osmolality*—a useful method of expressing the concentration of osmotically-active constituents of urine or any other solution. The osmotic pressure of a solution depends on the total number of particles (undissociated molecules and ions) per unit volume or mass of fluid and it is therefore convenient to use units which depend on the number of such particles present. For a substance which does not dissociate in solution, one osmole is a measure of the number of particles in 1 gramme-molecule, and a solution of 1 osmole/kg (or 1 gramme-molecule/kg) exerts an osmotic pressure of 22·4 atmospheres. If the molecules dissociate at all, the number of particles will increase and 1 gramme-molecule/kg will then exert a correspondingly higher osmotic pressure. For example, a solution of 1 gramme-molecule/kg of

FIG. 2. (a) Transverse section through a rabbit kidney, the blood vessels of which have been injected with Indian ink. Note the very numerous glomeruli in the cortex. C, cortex; SC, subcortex; O, outer medulla; I, inner medulla; P, pelvis of ureter; PAP, papilla. (b) Diagram of longitudinal section of human kidney, to show how the medullary substance is subdivided into a number of pyramids.

4

sodium chloride, which dissociates almost completely, has an osmolality of nearly 2 Osm/kg. For biological purposes, the osmole is too large a unit and the milliosmole (mOsm, one-thousandth of an osmole) is usually used. The concentration of osmotically-active particles in a solution may then be expressed in mOsm/kg water. An expert physicist would find this explanation somewhat oversimplified, but it will suffice for present purposes.

The osmolality of human blood plasma lies in the region of 300 mOsm/kg. Maximally concentrated urine may have an osmolality of 1400 mOsm/kg; it is 4 to 5 times as concentrated as plasma. In animals which live under arid conditions, even greater concentrations of urine can be obtained, the north African sand rat (*Psammomys*), for instance, being able to attain the astonishing level of 6000 mOsm/kg. This tiny animal can therefore concentrate its glomerular filtrate, which has an osmolality in the region of 300 mOsm/kg (equivalent to an osmotic pressure of about 7 atmospheres), to a final urine with an osmolality equivalent to an osmotic pressure of almost 140 atmospheres.

Such an enormous change in concentration cannot be brought about by simple reabsorption of water from the lumen of the tubules and it became necessary to seek another explanation for the concentrating power of the kidney. Since about 1950 the importance of the renal medulla has been recognized in this respect. Prior to this time, the medulla was thought to be a rather uninteresting and inactive region compared to the cortex and it was difficult to imagine any reason for the extraordinary course of the loops of Henle, which dip down for varying distances into the medulla before bending sharply back on themselves in a hairpin turn and returning to the cortex (Fig. 1). It is now known that the loops play an important part in producing a high osmolality in the tissues of the medulla which, in turn, is responsible for raising the osmolality of the final urine as it passes through the medulla in the collecting ducts.

The kidney is an organ in which structure and function are very closely correlated so that many

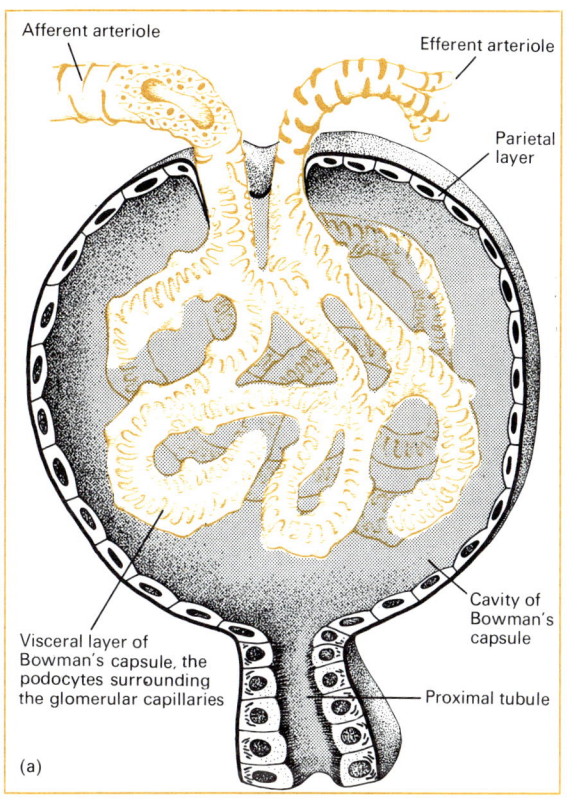

(a)

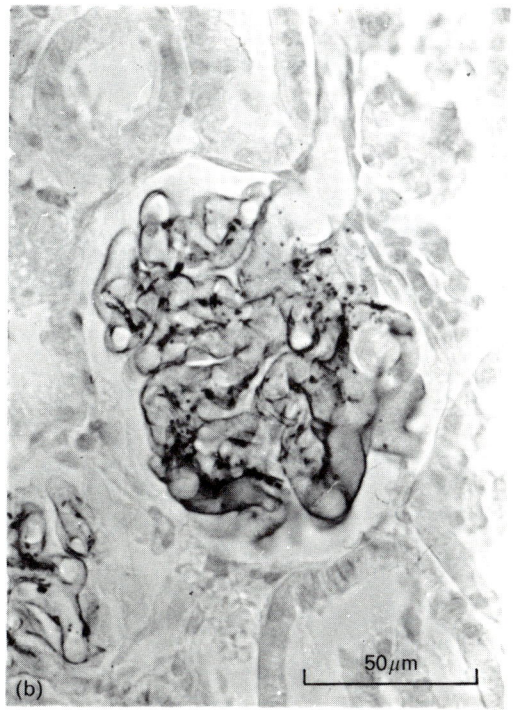

(b)

FIG. 3. (a) Diagram of Bowman's capsule and the glomerular tuft of capillaries. (b) Photomicrograph of a section of a glomerulus from a rat kidney. The section has not passed through the proximal tubule.

5

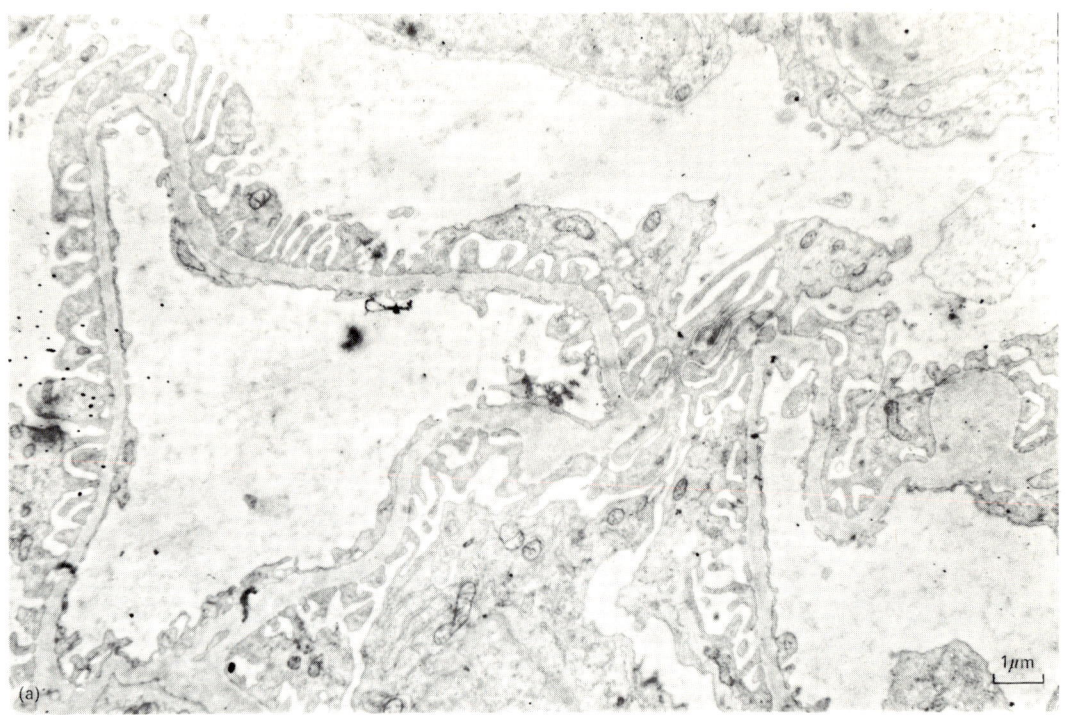

(a)

1μm

deductions about its functions can be made from a detailed study of its structure. In the account which follows, the arrangement and structure of the various components of the kidney will be described and an attempt made to explain the significance of their structure in functional terms.

The nephron

The *nephron*, the basic unit of the kidney, consists of a *glomerulus* and a long *tubule* in which a number of sharply demarcated segments can be distinguished (Fig. 1). Each glomerulus consists of a cluster of capillaries which invaginate the hollow blind end of a tubule, the thinned-out walls of which form the inner and outer layers of *Bowman's capsule*. The cavity of Bowman's capsule leads directly into the *proximal convoluted tubule* which, after a tortuous course, has a short, straight segment. The tubule then becomes smaller and its wall becomes thinner, as it passes down into the medulla for a varying distance to form the descending limb of the *loop of Henle*. Returning towards the cortex, the ascending limb abruptly becomes thick again, finally becoming the *distal convoluted tubule*. This opens into a *collecting duct*, along with a number of other distal tubules, which conveys the urine once more through the medulla

FIG. 4. (a) An electron micrograph of part of a glomerulus from a rat kidney, together with (b) a diagram of a possible arrangement of capillaries and cells in this specimen. Note how the foot processes of the epithelial cells inter-digitate so that a narrow winding slit-pore is left between them. The cut ends of the capillaries show that the glomerular filtrate has to pass through the endothelium, the basement membrane, and the slit-pore in order to reach Bowman's capsule. This is illustrated at a higher magnification in Fig. 5.

to empty into the pelvis of the ureter. In each human kidney there are roughly one million such nephrons.

The different portions of the nephron are so clearly demarcated that in an appropriately prepared transverse section the kidney can easily be seen to be subdivided into a number of zones, each of which contains particular segments of the nephron (Fig. 2). The outermost zone, the cortex, contains the glomeruli, the greater part of the proximal tubules, the distal tubules, and the beginning of the collecting ducts. Inside the cortex lies the subcortex, characterized particularly by the straight descending parts of the proximal tubules. The medulla is itself subdivided, the outer medulla containing the thin descending limbs of the loops of Henle, the thick ascending limbs and, of course, collecting ducts. The inner medulla

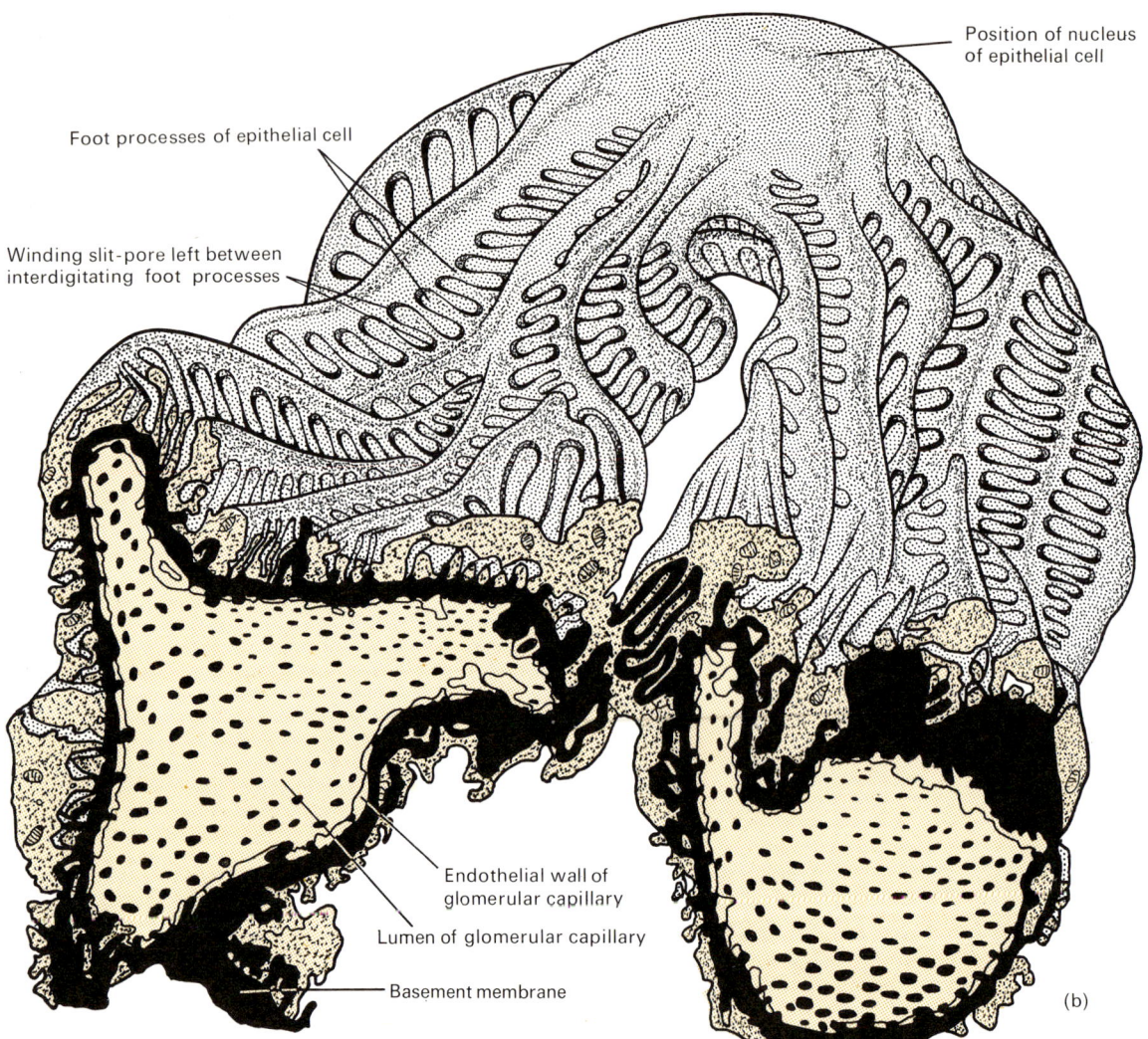

Position of nucleus
of epithelial cell

Foot processes of epithelial cell

Winding slit-pore left between
interdigitating foot processes

Endothelial wall of
glomerular capillary

Lumen of glomerular capillary

Basement membrane

(b)

contains the thin descending and thin ascending limbs of the loops of Henle and the larger collecting ducts. Blood vessels, including a rich capillary plexus, are found in each zone. The portion of the inner medulla which projects freely into the pelvis of the ureter is known as the papilla.

The structure of the human kidney (and that of some animals) is essentially similar to the rabbit (Fig. 2 (a)) but is a little more complex. The cortex forms a complete surface layer but the medullary substance is subdivided into a number of units known as renal pyramids (Fig. 2 (b)), each of which is similar to the medulla of the rabbit. The papillae of the pyramids project into subdivisions of the pelvis of the ureter which are called calyces (sing. calyx).

The glomerulus

The structure of the glomerulus is seen diagrammatically in Fig. 3, along with a photomicrograph. The afferent arteriole, which provides the blood supply to the glomerulus, breaks up to form a network of anastomosing capillaries which reunite to form the outgoing or efferent arteriole. In the majority of the glomeruli this is very short and soon branches to form a capillary network around the cortical tubules. A somewhat different arrangement is found in those glomeruli which lie nearest to the medulla (the *juxtamedullary glomeruli*) and this will be described later (p. 15). The glomerular capillaries themselves are closely surrounded by a layer of thin epithelial cells which form the inner, or visceral, layer of Bowman's

7

capsule. At the vascular pole of the glomerulus these inner cells are continuous with the outer or parietal layer, which in turn is continuous with the much taller epithelial cells of the proximal tubule.

The function of the glomerulus is to produce a practically protein-free ultrafiltrate of the blood plasma; this enters the cavity of Bowman's capsule and passes into the proximal tubule. Although the glomerular capillaries are permeable to many proteins with relatively low molecular weights, such as haemoglobin, they are almost completely impervious to the proteins which are normally present in blood plasma. The driving force behind the filtering process is the blood pressure within the capillaries, which is probably in the region of 70–75 mm Hg. Since, in many renal diseases, plasma proteins (especially albumin) may leak through into the glomerular filtrate, the structure of the barrier between blood and filtrate is of considerable importance and is worth examining in some detail.

It is first necessary to understand that while the cells of the outer layer of Bowman's capsule form a complete layer of flattened epithelium, those of the inner layer are of a much more complicated form, which is shown in Fig. 4. These cells, which are sometimes known as *podocytes* (literally 'foot-cells'), are similar to starfish in shape, the 'arms' or *trabeculae* each possessing a number of secondary or foot processes (*pedicels*). The cells are arranged so that their trabeculae and foot processes embrace one or more capillaries; the picture is made more complicated by the interdigitation of the foot processes with those of the adjacent cells (Fig. 5). The tortuous cleft between the meshed foot processes is known as the *slit-pore* since it is obvious that the glomerular filtrate has to percolate through this narrow cleft in order to reach the cavity of Bowman's capsule. In fact, the slit-pore is not an open space, for in a good electron-micrograph one can see that it is closed by a very thin membrane (Fig. 5). The capillaries themselves have a simple structure, consisting of an endothelium resting on a basement membrane. Except in the region of the nucleus, the endothelial cells are extremely thin and are perforated by large numbers of roughly circular openings or fenestrations which have a diameter of between 50 and 100 nm (Figs. 4, 5, and 6). Opinions differ as to the nature of the fenestrations. Some investigators have reported that they are not true pores since they are closed by a very thin membrane. This is certainly the case in the capillaries of other regions of the kidney (Fig. 14), but the majority opinion favours the view that no membrane is present in the glomerular capillaries; the apparent discrepancy in findings may well be due to species differences.

In passing from the capillary lumen to the cavity of Bowman's capsule, the glomerular filtrate must traverse (a) the endothelium, (b) the basement membrane, and (c) the slit-pores between the foot processes (Figs. 4 and 5). Somewhere within this composite membrane lies the physiological filtration system which allows some molecules to pass through but retains larger molecules such as proteins. In spite of the importance of this membrane and much intensive research, the exact mechanism of filtration remains unknown. A number of attempts have been made to investigate the problem by the injection into the bloodstream of animals of substances, such as colloidal iron, which are electron-opaque and which can therefore be seen in electron micrographs. The particles of these substances leave the glomerular capillaries and are found in the basement membrane and beyond it but are not always found in close relation to the fenestrations. Unfortunately, the electron microscope, in its present form, can only take a series of still photographs. Cine films are impossible to make so that the means whereby the particles pass through the endothelium is still uncertain. Some very convincing electron micrographs have, however, been published showing certain proteins apparently passing directly through the fenestrations and into the basement membrane (Karnovsky 1968). Current evidence indicates that the important filtering action takes place in the basement membrane, but its mechanism is not clearly understood and may not be identical for all substances.

The glomerular filtrate

The volume of filtrate produced by the glomeruli can be estimated by various indirect methods. The kidneys, between them, receive about one quarter of the total output of the heart, amounting to some 1300 cm³ of blood per minute in man. This blood contains about 700 cm³ of plasma (the rest of the volume is made up of cells) and of this, about 125 cm³ per minute is filtered off by the glomeruli. This amounts to a total daily filtrate of something like 180 litres. Under normal conditions,

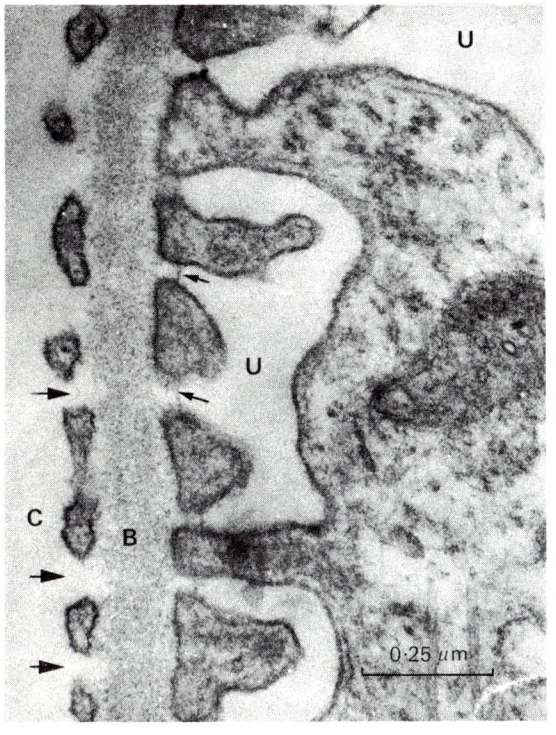

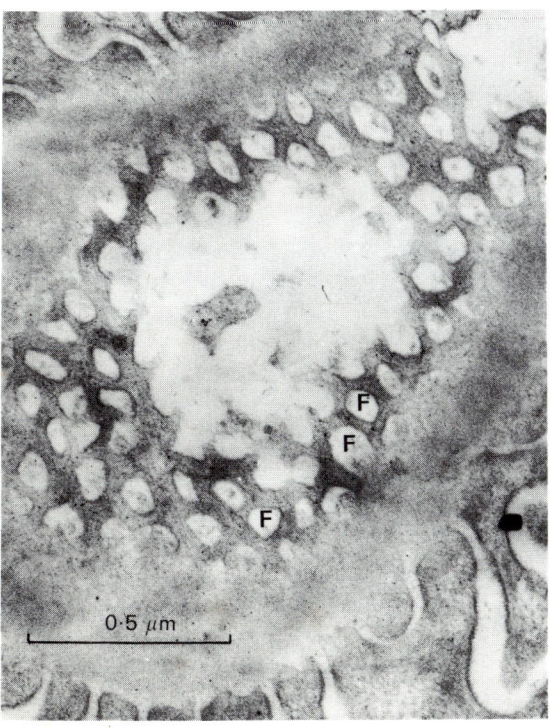

the volume of urine produced is only in the region of 1·5 l, so that about 178·5 l of filtrate is (fortunately) reabsorbed by the tubules of the kidney. If one studies this reabsorption of water in detail, one finds that the greater part of the 125 cm³ of filtrate which is produced each minute is reabsorbed by the proximal tubule, leaving only 15–20 cm³/min to pass into the loops of Henle. This proximal tubule reabsorption is relatively constant and is therefore sometimes known as the 'obligatory reabsorption'. The remaining 20 cm³/min is reabsorbed to a varying extent ('facultative reabsorption') so that the final volume of urine varies between 0·3 cm³ and 20 cm³/min. These figures are approximate and may vary considerably between individuals.

Obligatory reabsorption in the proximal tubule
The study of the functions of the renal tubules has been greatly facilitated by the technique of micropuncture in which, by means of a micromanipulator, extremely fine hollow glass needles may be used to withdraw fluid from the tubules and blood vessels of the kidney or to inject various foreign substances, the fate of which may then be determined. This technique was first applied to the mammalian kidney by Walker and his colleagues in 1941. An excellent account of the methods used and the results obtained has been given by Windhager (1968). Experiments of this kind showed that in the proximal tubule, the reabsorption of water is apparently secondary to the active reabsorption of sodium. Sodium is reabsorbed by the cells and passed into the capillaries, accompanied by appropriate anions (principally chloride) and also accompanied by an equivalent amount of water to maintain the osmotic equilibrium. Various other substances such as glucose are reabsorbed in the proximal tubule but the fluid remains iso-osmotic (i.e. having the same osmolality) with respect to plasma so that no concentration or dilution of the tubular fluid occurs in this region. Of course, not all the

FIG. 5. The membrane between the blood and the cavity of Bowman's capsule. The lumen of the capillary (C) lies to the left; the cavity of Bowman's capsule (U) to the right. The endothelium has numerous fenestrations (large arrows). The slit-pores between the foot processes are closed by a thin membrane (small arrows). The principal structure separating blood from glomerular filtrate is the basement membrane (B).
FIG. 6. A tangential section through a glomerular capillary. The endothelial fenestrations are clearly visible (F).

sodium or water in the proximal tubule is re-absorbed or the output of urine would come to a standstill, but the mechanism whereby the amount of reabsorption is regulated is not known although there are a number of theories. This interesting problem has recently been discussed by Dicker (1970).

The structure of the proximal tubule reveals something of its functions: the cells show several features which are characteristic of cells which transport large quantities of salts and water. The surface which faces the lumen of the tubule has a brush border which can easily be seen when an appropriate stain is used (Fig. 7 (a)). Electron microscopy shows the brush border to consist of a large number of microvilli (Fig. 8) which enor-mously increase the surface area of the cell. Between the bases of the microvilli are found small and large vesicles which are engaged in absorption from the lumen of the tubule. The energy required for active transport is provided by the enzyme activity of the numerous mitochondria which are present in the cells. The outermost or basal surface of the cell also shows very complex infoldings of the cell membrane, another device which increases the surface area. Basal infoldings are also a feature of the cells of most of the other kidney tubules and are particularly well seen in the thick ascending limb of Henle's loop (Fig. 11 (b)).

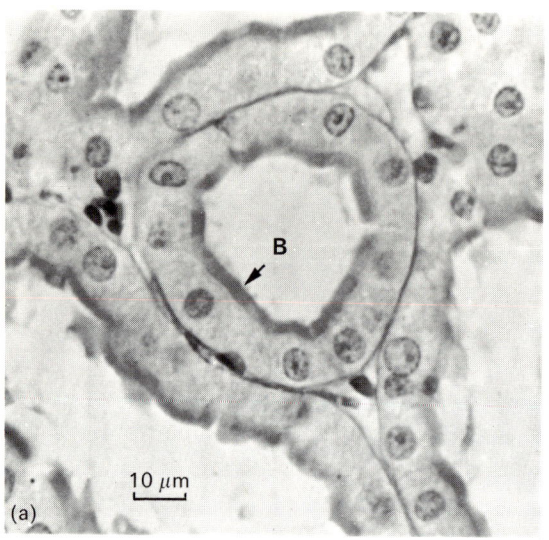

10 μm

(a)

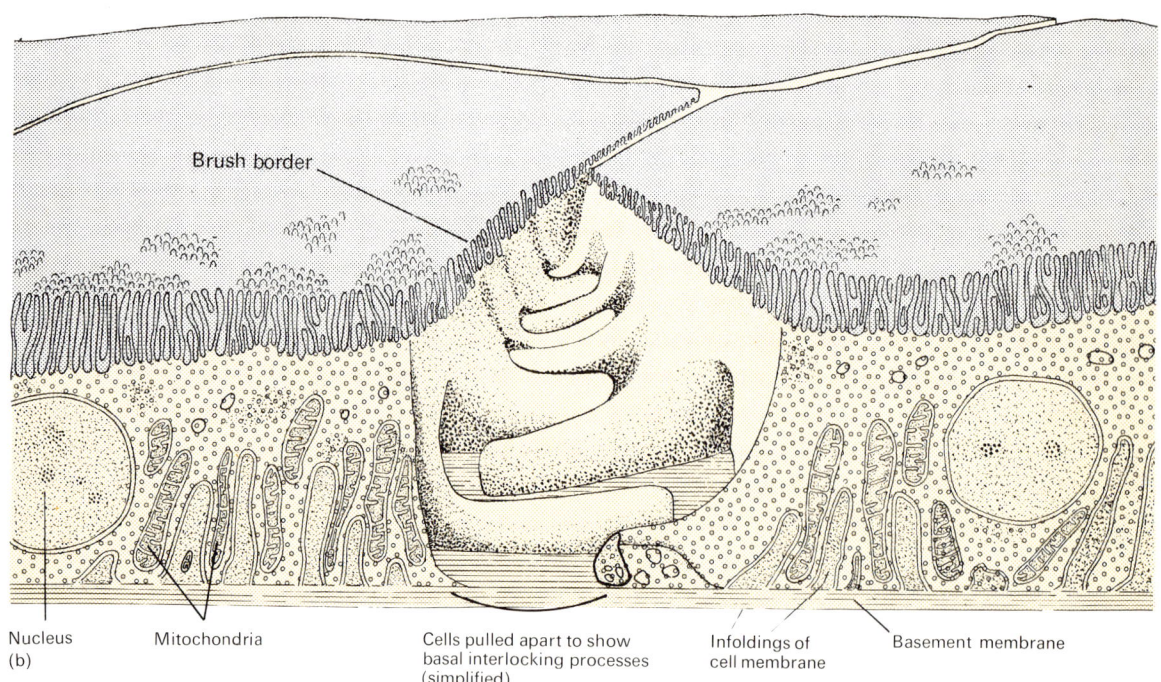

Brush border

Nucleus
(b)

Mitochondria

Cells pulled apart to show basal interlocking processes (simplified)

Infoldings of cell membrane

Basement membrane

FIG. 7. (a) Transverse section through a proximal tubule stained by the periodic acid-Schiff technique to show the brush border (B). (b) Drawing of the shapes and interdigitations of the cells of the proximal convoluted tubule.

Facultative reabsorption in the distal part of the nephron

Earlier theories about the concentration of urine by the gradual reabsorption of water as the glomerular filtrate passes along the tubules became more and more difficult to accept in the light of experimental results. For example, micropuncture studies by Walker and his colleagues indicated that the tubular fluid at the beginning of the distal tubule of the rat is usually hypo-osmotic (i.e. it has an osmolality below that of plasma). Another important finding was that of Wirz, Hargitay, and Kuhn in 1951 who investigated the osmolality of rat renal medulla by utilizing the principle that the osmolality of a solution is closely related to its freezing point. The technique actually used was to find the thawing point of previously frozen slices of kidney, and these experiments showed that there is an osmotic gradient in the tissues of the medulla, increasing towards the tip where osmolality is up to 8 times that of plasma. The osmolality of all structures at any one level in the medulla is approximately equal. Putting these findings together, it seems that the iso-osmotic fluid leaving the proximal tubule becomes more and more concentrated as it descends the loop of Henle but then becomes less and less concentrated again as it ascends until, as it enters the distal tubule, it is hypo-osmotic. Further clues to the functions of the loop of Henle came from comparative studies. Only birds and mammals are able to produce a concentrated urine and only they possess a complete Henle's loop. There is also a correlation between the relative thickness of the medulla in different species (Fig. 9) and the ability to produce concentrated urine (Schmidt-Nielsen and O'Dell 1961).

These observations, viewed in isolation, seem to be very puzzling but a theory which fits all the facts had already been advanced before most of them had been made. In 1942, Kuhn and Ryffel suggested that a counter-current multiplication process, already familiar to physicists, might be applicable to the kidney. This idea is now generally accepted, with some modifications, and current research work is largely concerned with determining the exact site and mechanism of the multiplier system.

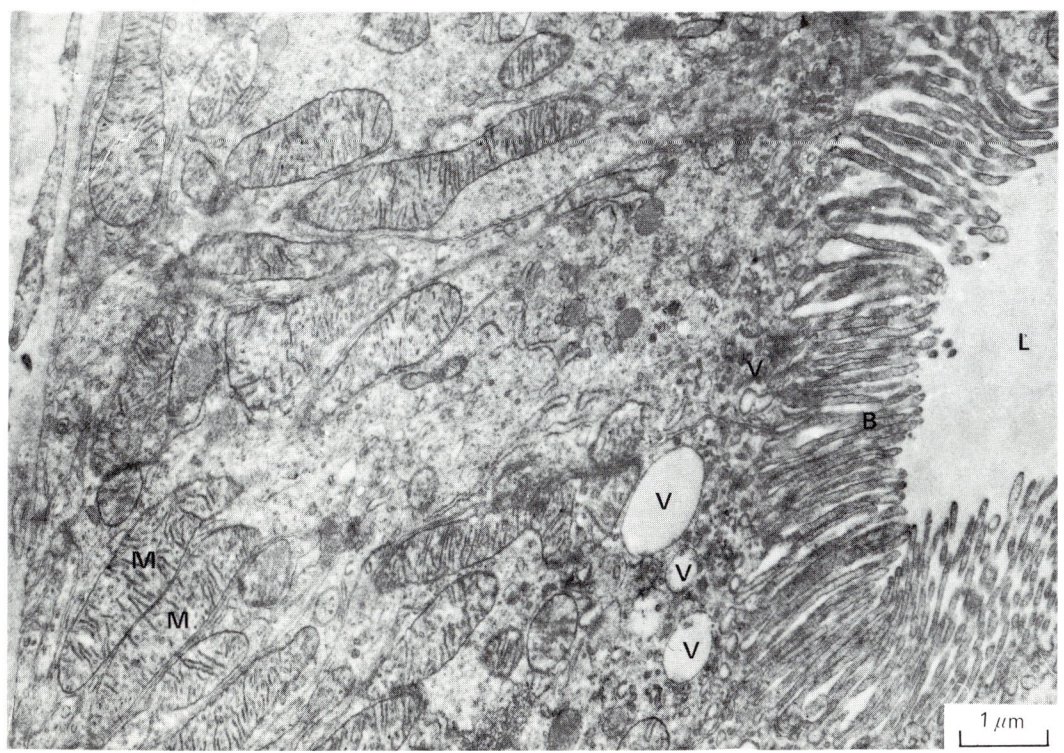

Fig. 8. Electron micrograph of a proximal tubule. The lumen (L) lies to the right. The brush border is composed of numerous microvilli (B). Note the large and small vesicles (V) and the abundant mitochondria (M).

11

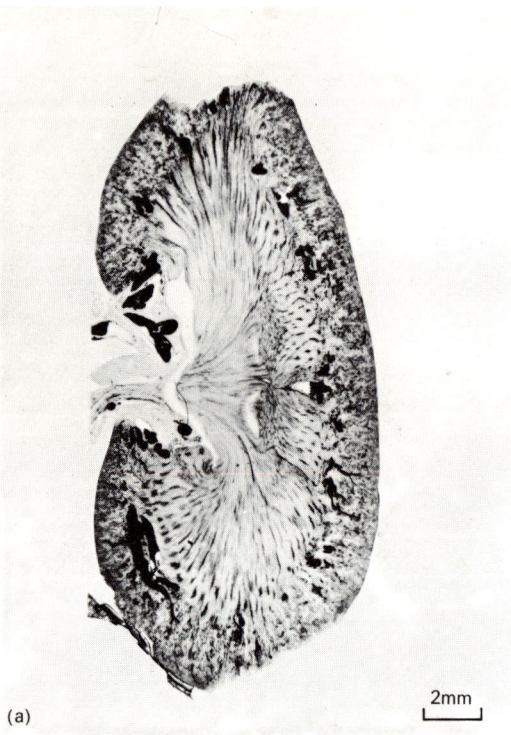

(a)

2mm

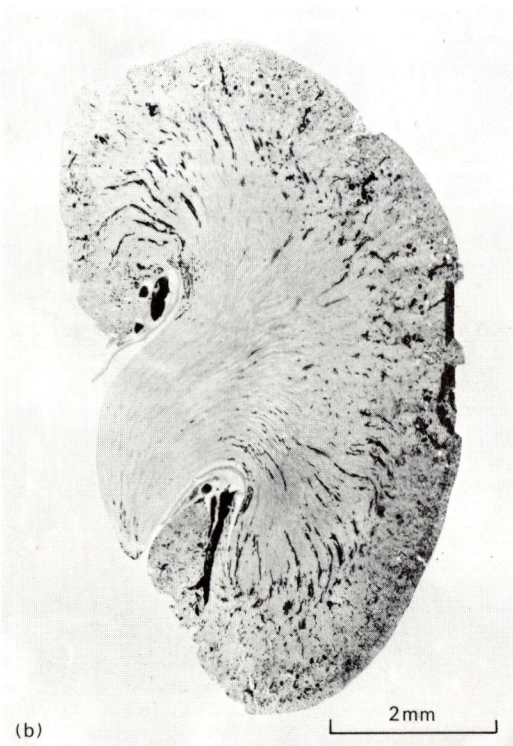

(b)

2mm

The principle of counter-current exchange and multiplication

A simple counter-current exchange system is illustrated by the engineer's method of using hot exhaust gas from an engine to heat the incoming air (Fig. 10). The gas, as it leaves the engine, is extremely hot, but as it passes along the exhaust tube it rapidly becomes cooler as heat is transferred to the incoming air which is flowing in the opposite direction (hence the use of the term 'counter-current'). The incoming air therefore becomes hotter as it approaches the engine. There is thus established a gradient of temperature in which the gas or air in both inlet and exhaust pipes is very hot near to the engine but is almost at atmospheric temperature near to the external apertures. Heat is thus not dissipated unto the atmosphere, but is conserved within the machine. Supposing that, for some extraordinary reason, the exhaust pipe were connected to the inlet pipe (Fig. 10(b)). Conditions, at least as far as the temperature in the tubes is concerned, would not be greatly altered. The cool gas, which previously escaped into the air, would now re-enter the machine, and would be re-heated in the process. This would not be a good idea for engines, but the same principle—that of a counter-current *exchanger*—is found in many biological situations. In aquatic mammals such as whales, for instance, the warm blood passing into the extremities would dissipate an enormous amount of the body heat into the Arctic seas were it not for the fact that the main artery of supply to the limb or flipper is very closely surrounded by a large number of veins which return the blood to the trunk. Heat is transferred from the artery to the veins along their length so that heat is conserved at the body end of the system.

In these heat counter-current exchange systems, the exchange of heat between the tubes is a passive or 'downhill' transfer down a heat gradient; such a system can only conserve the heat which is already present—it cannot build up extra heat. Fig. 10(c) shows a further development of the counter-current principle in which an active or 'uphill' transport system takes part. The U-tube is supposed to

FIG. 9. Longitudinal sections of the kidneys of (a) a ferret and (b) a steppe lemming. The latter is an animal which can concentrate its urine to a very high degree. Note how its inner medulla is so long that it projects into the ureter.

contain a circulating sodium chloride solution and a mechanism is present which is capable of *actively* transferring sodium (and chloride) ions from the ascending to the descending limb of the U-tube, without any accompanying water. As a result of this process the osmolality of the fluid in the descending limb will increase as it approaches the hairpin bend. After rounding the bend, the highly concentrated fluid will gradually undergo a diminution in osmolality as solute is extruded (without water) until the fluid emerges from the upper end of the tube with an osmolality slightly below that at which it entered the system. When *active* transport occurs, therefore, if the loop is long enough, a very high osmolality can be built up towards the U-bend although at any one level only a small osmotic gradient exists between the two tubes. Thus the 'single effect' of a small active transfer of solute at any one level can be multiplied along the length of the tube to produce a large total effect and this is therefore known as a counter-current *multiplier* system. Active transport of sodium ions is sometimes referred to as the 'sodium pump' and it requires the expenditure of energy.

Counter-current multiplication in the loops of Henle
This process, with some modification, forms the basis for the establishment of the osmotic gradient in the medulla of the kidney and the figures for osmolality which are shown in Fig. 10 (c) might apply to a loop of Henle. In the loops, sodium, along with appropriate anions (mostly chloride), is actively transported out of the ascending limb into the interstitial (intertubular) tissue and then into the descending limb so that a multiplier system is set up and the osmolality of the loops of Henle and the interstitial tissue (including the blood vessels) increases towards the tip of the papilla. The collecting ducts have to travel through this zone of greatly increased osmolality in order to pass their contents into the pelvis of the ureter (Fig. 1) and a mechanism can now be envisaged which will allow for the production of a concentrated or a diluted urine as the situation demands. If the walls of the collecting ducts were water-permeable, water would leave the ducts to pass into the hyperosmotic surroundings so that the final urine would become relatively concentrated. If, on the other hand, the walls were impermeable, the hypoosmotic fluid from the distal tubule would be led by the collecting ducts safely through their hyperosmotic surroundings without any loss of water so that the urine would remain dilute. The permeability of the collecting ducts is controlled by the anti-diuretic hormone (ADH). The excretion of a large amount of dilute urine is known as *diuresis* and the *anti*-diuretic hormone, which is secreted by the pituitary gland in response to the need for conserving water, leads to the production of a concentrated urine by increasing the permeability of the collecting ducts. The permeability of the distal tubule to water is also increased by ADH and when sodium is reabsorbed in this part of the nephron an osmotically equivalent amount of water accompanies it, thus contributing towards

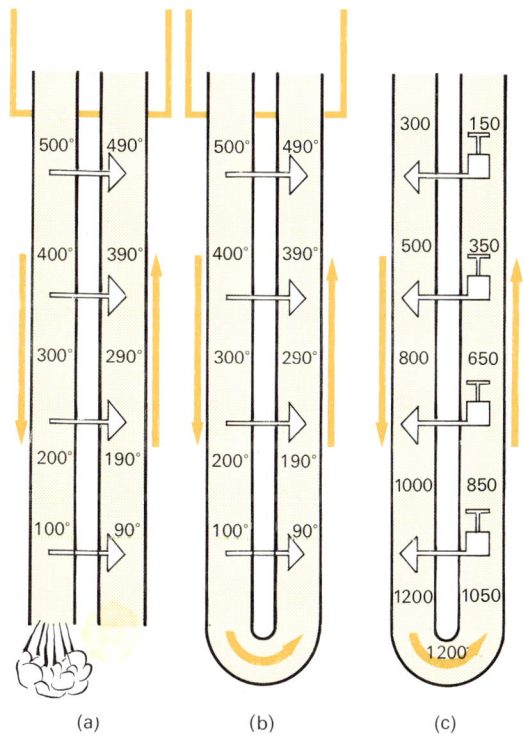

(a)   (b)   (c)

FIG. 10. Diagrams to represent (a) heating of incoming air by exhaust gas in an engine; in practice a large number of tubes are used to increase the surface area available for heat exchange; (b) a counter-current heat-exchange system; and (c) a counter-current *multiplier* system involving the *active* transport of sodium from the ascending limb to the descending limb, by means of a 'sodium pump'. This has the effect of building up a high osmolality (expressed in mOsm/kg) towards the U-bend although at any one level there is only a small difference in osmolality between the two limbs.

the concentration of fluid in the tubules.

To sum up, the large volume of glomerular filtrate is reduced by roughly 80% by the active reabsorption of sodium, accompanied by an osmotically equivalent amount of water. A relatively small volume of iso-osmotic fluid enters the loop of Henle and it leaves the loop as a hypo-osmotic solution. During its passage through the loop it has established an osmotic gradient in the medulla by a counter-current multiplier system involving the active transport of sodium (and chloride) ions from the ascending limb, to the descending limb. More sodium is reabsorbed from the distal tubule and the fluid then traverses the hyperosmotic medulla in the collecting duct. If ADH is present water accompanies sodium out of the distal tubule and also is osmotically withdrawn from the collecting duct as it passes through the hyperosmotic medulla; this produces a concentrated urine. In the absence of ADH, water remains in the distal tubule and in the collecting duct since the walls are impermeable to water. The urine is then dilute.

The above account is very dogmatic and simplified. The mechanisms involved are much more complicated and controversial than appears here. While the general principle of counter-current multiplication by the loops of Henle is almost universally accepted, many different views have been put forward as to how, exactly, the process occurs. For example, it is not necessary for the function of the counter-current mechanism that the sodium reabsorbed from the ascending limb of Henle's loop should actually pass into the descending limb. If it stays in the interstitial tissue between the tubules and the consequent increase in osmolality causes withdrawal of water without solute from the descending limb, the final result would be the same.

In order to set up any form of counter-current system, the properties of the ascending and descending limbs have to be very different with regard to the transport of sodium and of water. The electron microscope, however, shows only minor structural differences, at least in the inner medulla. Another difficulty is that the structure of the thin limbs of the loop is relatively simple and they contain only a few mitochondria (Fig. 11 (a)). This does not suggest that the thin ascending limb is adapted for active sodium transport, which requires the expenditure of energy. The thick part of the ascending limb looks much more promising as a 'sodium pump' (Fig. 11 (b)). It contains numerous mitochondria and the cell membrane at the base of the cell shows the extremely complicated deep infoldings which are characteristic of cells in

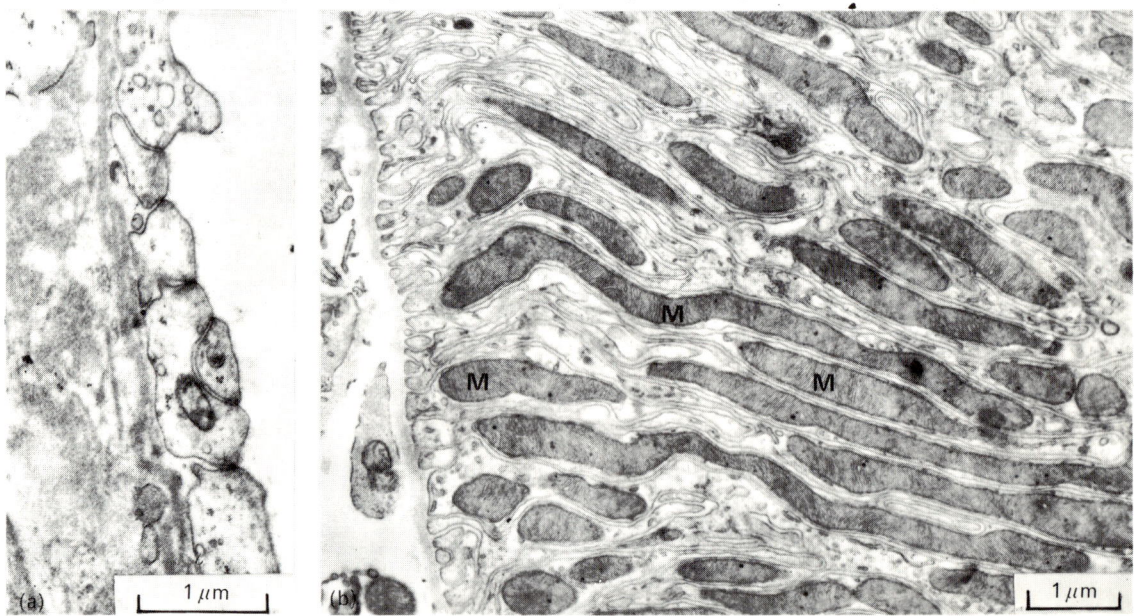

FIG. 11. (a) Thin segment of Henle's loop from the inner medulla. The lumen lies to the right. (b) Part of the thick ascending limb of Henle's loop from the outer medulla. Note the deep infoldings of the cell membrane at the base of the cell which lies to the left. This brings the membrane very close to the numerous mitochondria (M).

14

which the transport of large quantities of fluid and salt occur. A number of workers have therefore suggested that sodium transport takes place only in the thick ascending limbs in the outer medulla. However, micropuncture experiments by Jamison and his colleagues (1967) have given important though not absolutely decisive evidence of counter-current multiplication in the thin limbs. A summary of the most up-to-date views on this subject is given in the papers presented at a recent symposium on medullary function, edited by Thurau (1970).

The medullary blood vessels

It is probable that counter-current multiplication in the loops of Henle is not the only factor concerned in building up and maintaining the osmotic gradient of the medulla. The anatomical peculiarities of the blood supply to the medulla suggest that the blood vessels may play an important part. The efferent arterioles of the glomeruli nearest to the medulla—the juxtamedullary glomeruli—have a course different from that of the efferent arterioles of the more superficial glomeruli. After leaving the glomerulus the efferent arteriole passes into the medulla and breaks up into a leash of vessels known as descending vasa recta (Figs. 12 and 13). These supply capillary networks in the medulla and from the capillaries, ascending vasa recta pass back towards the cortex where they join some of the larger veins (Fourman and Moffat 1964). In the outer medulla, the descending and ascending vasa recta are gathered together to form vascular bundles in which the two types of vessel are intermingled and come into close apposition (Fig. 13). Electron microscopy shows that in the bundles the ascending and descending vessels are separated by no more than a very thin layer of interstitial tissue and at most, the thickness of only one cell lies between them (Fig. 14). Structurally, this arrangement is obviously well suited to a counter-current mechanism. It has been suggested that the hydrostatic pressure in the descending vasa recta may provide the driving force for a multiplication mechanism by the active transport of water, but this view is not widely held,

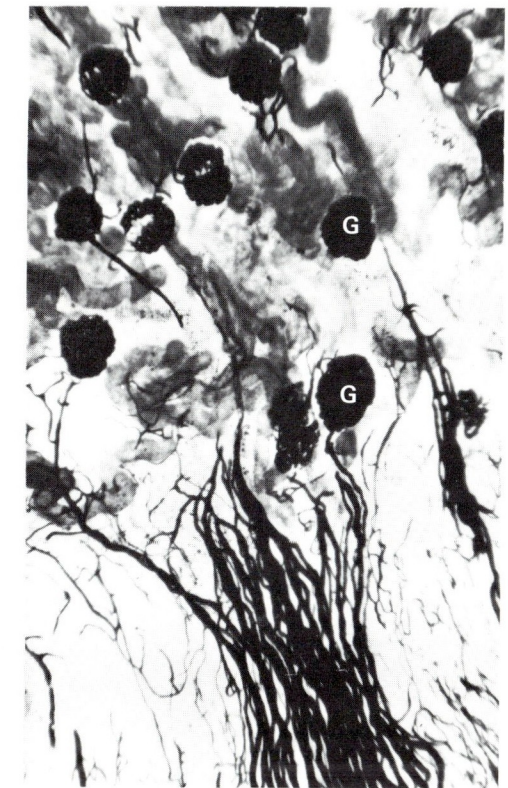

FIG. 12. Juxtamedullary glomeruli (G) whose efferent arterioles break up into bundles of descending vasa recta. The vessels have been injected with Indian ink.

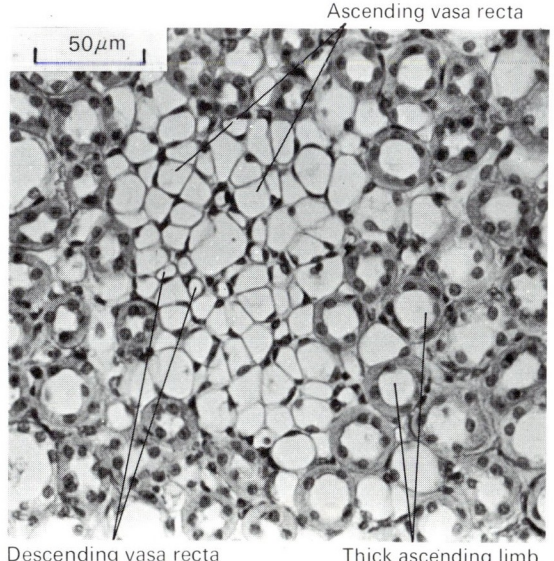

Ascending vasa recta

50 μm

Descending vasa recta

Thick ascending limb of loop of Henle

FIG. 13. Transverse section through a vascular bundle of the rat kidney. The smaller vessels are descending vasa recta while the larger are ascending vasa recta (with a few thin loops of Henle). The thick-walled structures which surround the bundle are thick ascending limbs of Henle's loops and collecting ducts.

15

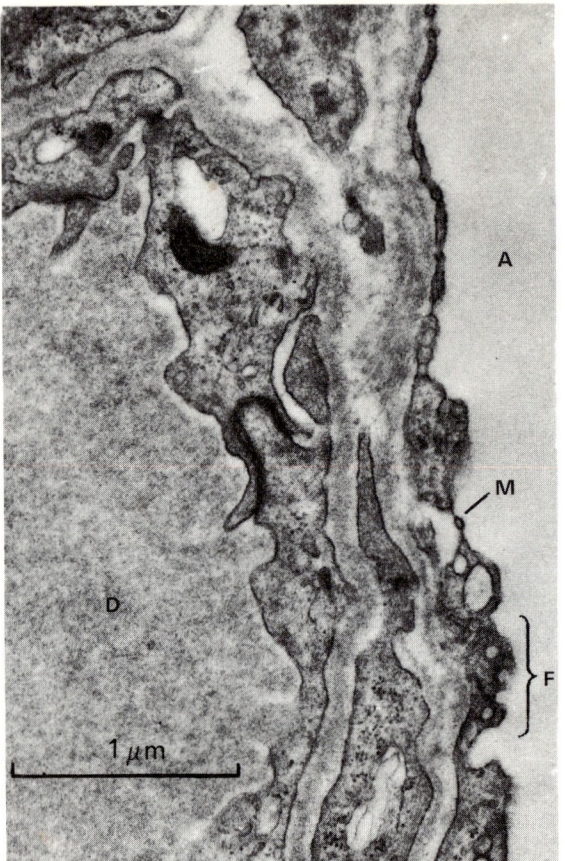

FIG. 14. Descending (D) and ascending (A) vasa recta from a vascular bundle. The former has a relatively thick endothelium but the latter is fenestrated. The fenestrations can be seen in tangential section at F and in profile at M, where it can be seen that they are closed by a membrane.

up a whole new field of investigation, much of which is still in its early stages. The metabolism of the renal medulla is peculiar, since this part of the kidney, for various reasons, operates at a very low oxygen tension and there is evidence for the importance of both aerobic and anaerobic metabolism. The precise mechanism whereby **ADH** increases the permeability of the distal part of the nephron to water is another matter for discussion. While the general idea of counter-current multiplication is accepted as the mechanism by which the kidney succeeds in its task of producing, when necessary, a highly concentrated urine, there is still an enormous amount of work to be done by morphologists, physiologists, and biochemists before this aspect of kidney function can be fully understood.

FURTHER READING

General

DALTON, A. J. and HAGUENAU, F. (1967). *Ultrastructure of the kidney*. Academic Press, New York.

DICKER, S. E. (1970). *Mechanisms of urine concentration and dilution in mammals*. Edward Arnold, London.

PITTS, R. F. (1968). *Physiology of the kidney and body fluids*. 2nd. edn. Year Book Medical Publishers Inc., Chicago.

For reference

FOURMAN, J. and MOFFAT, D. B. (1964). Observations on the fine blood vessels of the kidney. *Symp. zool. Soc. Lond.* **11**, 57–71.

JAMISON, R. L., BENNETT, C. M., and BERLINER, R. W. (1967). Counter-current multiplication by the thin loops of Henle. *Am. J. Physiol.* **212**, 352–66.

KARNOVSKY, M. J. (1968). The ultrastructural basis of transcapillary permeability. *J. gen. Physiol.* **52**, 64S–95S.

SCHMIDT-NIELSEN, B. and O'DELL, R. (1961). Structure and concentrating mechanism in the mammalian kidney. *Am. J. Physiol.* **200**, 1119–24.

THURAU, K. (ed.) (1970). Symposium on renal medullary function. *Proc. IV Int. Congr. Nephrol.*, 136–74.

WALKER, A., BOTT, P., OLIVER, J., and MACDOWELL, M. C. (1941). The collection and analysis of fluid from single nephrons of the mammalian kidney. *Am. J. Physiol.* **134**, 580–95.

WINDHAGER, E. E. (1968). *Micropuncture techniques and nephron function*. Butterworth, London.

though most workers believe that one or more counter-current exchange systems occur in this region. For example, the diffusion of water from descending to ascending limb would exclude a quantity of water from the medulla and thus assist in maintaining the osmotic gradient, without actually being responsible for it.

There are many other interesting aspects of the physiology and anatomy of the concentrating mechanism of the kidney which need to be discussed but it will only be possible to mention some of them briefly in this account. There is little doubt that part of the osmotic gradient in the medulla is due to urea and there is evidence that this substance, as well as sodium, takes part in a counter-current mechanism. The excretion of water is closely bound up with that of salt, but this opens